FINDING THE GOOD DURING BAD TIMES WITH MULTIPLE SCLEROSIS

Multiple Sclerosis is a downright horrible disease to have to live with. You have to face many different challenges throughout the years. Eating right, exercising, and sleeping well are just some of the ways that you can take care of yourself along with finding a disease modifying medication that will help to relieve some of the many symptoms that are caused by MS. This book is about my personal journey over the past 14 years as I struggled with the progression of the disease and finding ways to stay active, healthy and continue to have a smile on my face.

Contents

MS Craziness

MY DIAGNOSIS

TREMORS

DOING THINGS DIFFERENTLY

SHAME AND DEPENDENCE

NEEDING A WHEELCHAIR

FATIGUE

COGNITIVE

IDENTITY

MEDICATIONS

LDN

EXERCISE

NUTRITION AND SUPPLEMENTS

SLEEP
INTERNET CAN HELP
DOCTOR'S APPOINTMENTS
HANDICAP PARKING
PROLOGUE

Thanks to my lovely wife, our great children, and our wonderful family for all your help and support. I wouldn't be where I am today without you.

MS Craziness

After thirteen years of trying a number of different medications to treat my multiple sclerosis (MS), I have finally found one that works wonders for me when taken with my ampyra and gilenya. Everyone is so happy and astonished with my improvements. Low dose naltrexone (LDN) is gradually helping me get out of the darkness that MS has so rudely and abruptly put me in for so many years. LDN is another piece of important medications that has been missing from the puzzle of MS treatment for too long. I feel that I'm running on three cylinders out of four now, instead of one and a half, or maybe two, depending on how the weather is.

It feels as though I have been so far down the rabbit hole that climbing out of it is simply not a walk in the park, so to speak. It takes a lot of hard work and dedication to improve yourself, but it's worth every minute of it. Every little achievement I make is another step closer to the end of that deep and dark rabbit hole I have been forced to live in for so many years. I am now able to see more and more light. I am even able to be in the sunlight on hot and humid days now. My quality of life has gotten better, and everyone notices it, including my doctors. You surely don't know all the pleasures of what you got until it's gone and you can't use it anymore.

Having MS has directly and sadly caused me to sit on the couch and fall asleep so many times. In fact, too many times in my book. It's really sad how much fatigue can play such a huge factor in the life of someone with MS. It feels as though if it's not one thing causing you to feel tired, then it's another. Even certain medications can make you tired and sleepy. It's like a catch 22, because you want to feel as good as you possibly can, but at the same time, you don't want to feel so tired from the medication you just took, and sleep yet another day away. Life goes by way too quickly, and I feel as though it's important and wise to keep moving and not to sleep your life away, so adding LDN to my other two medications really helped me not sleep all day, and actually be able to help out a lot more in the house.

A very important thing to remember is the fact that having MS does not only affect the individual with the awful disease, but also your spouse, your entire family, and friends, as well.

So many plans and activities may very well have to be rethought, or even canceled throughout the day and week. You think about what handy device do I need to use today to help me get from point A to point B, both inside and outside of places? How many steps will I have to climb? Will there be an elevator? Will there be a ramp? Will there be a restroom close by? What is the weather currently like now and what is the prediction, or forecast for later? Let's hope the prediction is correct, because that will greatly change things if it's not. We would not want to be caught outside in a storm, for so many different reasons. One reason in particular is the fact that I would not be able to move quickly using my cane and having my neurotransmitters in my body try to get messages across damaged pathways. Me and quick just do not get along. Hopefully, we will one day, and what a fine day it would be, too. Until that day arrives, anyone with me in the meantime will most likely get soaked, as well, because I feel like I move like a sloth at times. When I try to rush, then absolute chaos is easily created and situations go downhill very quickly.

    Meanwhile, I have to make sure I don't walk on wet floors with my cane, or the pegs on my cane will get wet, and I will easily slip and fall. Trust me, I have had it happen to me a number of times, and I'm sure it has happened to many of you, as well. Some of these wet areas that I have to be more aware of are near water fountains in stores and mopped floors. Using a cane on these wet surfaces can easily make my cane slip, thus making me unstable and more apt to fall. This is never a good thing. So many different types of injury can occur in this circumstance and nobody wants that, at least nobody I know, including me.

Sometimes the weather determines what type of day or night I will have. Such nasty weather for me includes heat and humidity. Before I started taking LDN, along with my other medications, heat and humidity would be lights out for me. I would be so fatigued that doing anything seemed very taxing on my body and impossible. A good analogy is superman with kryptonite close by. Heat and humidity just sucked all of my energy and strength directly out of my body. Zap, you're done for this day, and most likely the following day, as well.

To put this another way, so many times I would have to watch my wife play with our children from looking out of the window. Many times they would play or do something outside while I was fast asleep inside on the bed with an air conditioner on cooling me down. I can't explain enough how much I wished I could be out there playing with them and having a grand ol time together. However, at least they had a great time all in all. I'm so happy about that, I just wish I could of been included, and outside in the heat and humidity, but this disease has other plans.

    I struggle getting from one place to another due to my poor balance, weak leg muscles, drop foot, and damaged pathways within my body. There have been many times when I have had to be helped up after falling from my wife and children, other family members, and even people I have never seen before in my life. It is said that I fall gracefully, so thank God. Maybe it's from my basketball years and me always trying to stay in the air for that extra split second and scoring while coming down rather softly to avoid getting hurt. Who knows!

One amazing and innovative piece of equipment that I have been able to use is called the walkaide. This device helps prevent my foot from dropping and hitting the ground, thus leading to me tripping and falling. This brace has electrodes connected to it that go on my calf and triggers my neurotransmitters to send a message to have my foot lift up at exactly the right time. It feels amazing to have my foot lift up with every step I take, even if it's hot and humid, thanks to a double

AA battery and great innovation from brilliant people for designing this amazing equipment for individuals that need it. With this brace on, I am not even required to wear shoes, so I am able to walk barefoot along the beach if I want to. I would usually carry an extra battery with me in case I heard the beeping alarm go off to let me know the battery was running low and needed to be changed. I once thought the low battery alarm was the smoke alarm inside the house when I was with my youngest son. No matter where I went in the house, I would hear the beeping noise. It finally dawned on me that the beeping noises were coming from my walkaide, and not a smoke alarm. That was a very silly moment for me. I was going crazy going from one room to another checking the different smoke alarms.

As many of us MSers and our caregivers are well aware of, heat and humidity play a big role in MS symptoms. Ergo, having foot drop is even more prevalent, so it's nice to have something help prevent your foot drop from occurring, in the first place. It's more than worth the battle we had with the insurance company in order to be approved for it and the money we had to raise in a small community and spend to get it. Good thing for friends and donations. My wife even had to have a friend write a letter explaining how well this walkaide worked for me to the insurance company. My physician's assistant (PA) had to also convince the insurance company that it worked well and made a positive difference for me with my gaite. What a battle that all was, but it's so nice when everyone comes together to help fight the insurance company, because numbers makes a difference. Sometimes the more people you have, then the stronger you are and the more apt you are winning your case against a big insurance company.

    Another common challenge many MSers have is spasticity. Certain types of this spasticity can easily cause your leg and foot not to be able to lift up as high as normal. Obviously, this negatively affects the way you walk during the day and night. As if you didn't already have enough problems and challenges in your life to think about. Well, you can take medicine called baclofen to help fight this feeling of spasticity go away, or mitigate it, but there is a chance of it causing you to feel tired. There is also a baclofen pump that can be surgically implanted in your back, as well. It's one of many choices you have to make. What works better for you, and what makes you happier? These are some of the many questions you should ask yourself beforehand. You want to make sure you are aware of the procedure before you have it done.

    I hate to have to bring this up, but when you get the sudden urge to urinate and at the same time can't hold it, then you end up having an accident in your clothes, because the floodgates open and there is no way you can stop it. What an embarrassing disaster! In fact, one way you know you have MS is that you have to make sure you know where all the restrooms are in all the places you go to and all the places in between. This is surely a moment with MS when your pride is stripped away from you, if you happen to have a much unwanted accident. Unfortunately, this can happen anywhere, even at a family gathering or a friend's house. This is what happens when you have a neurogenic bladder. As usual, you will experience good and not so good days.

One important lesson to learn is that you should try to train your bladder to void every two hours, even if you don't feel the urge. Another great idea is not to drink anything two hours before you go to an event, if you can, and to void right before you leave. An awful mistake you can make is to not try to use the restroom. It may sound silly, but I'm absolutely sure many of you know what I'm talking about. Something else to avoid is having coffee before you have to leave to go somewhere, because oftentimes this will affect your bladder and give you a feeling of urgency and frequency. Fortunately, my wife suggested a caffeine pill in these circumstances in order to avoid drinking coffee and to also avoid getting a real bad headache from not having my cup of caffeine juice, or much better known as coffee.

Although these tips are helpful, there is no guarantee that it will help and prevent you from having an accident all of the time. There are days you constantly feel the urge to urinate. I like to call these days "the day of the bladder," because it seems like that's going to be a day you have to use the restroom a lot more than usual. There are other days that go by without the sudden and frequent urge to urinate all the time. Let's hope you have to go out to a doctor's appointment, or a family event, on a nice day when you don't have that frequent and sudden urge.

It is true that some people have to wear depends, or an adult diaper, and still others may have to go around with a catheter and bag if medications don't help that the urologist, neurologist, or family doctor, prescribed. This is all a part of MS that happens to so many of us that suffer from this crazy and downright cruel disease. There is even a chance someone needs a bag, or stoma, to hold their poop, as well. Some people have two bags, one for each of their bathroom needs. MS can just be that crazy, unfortunately.

There happens to be a very good reason why many different people call us "MS Warriors," but let's not forget that caregivers are warriors, as well.

Yet another crazy feeling many MSers have, and often times go through, is this itching feeling that seems to be right under the skin, and impossible to satisfy by scratching. It can drive many people bazerk, because you can't satisfy the itch at all, and it just lingers for however long it decides to. Sometimes the unforgiving itch can last for minutes and then go away, but come right back again within a minute or two. Did I mention how irritating this can be?

There are other times when that irritating itch under the skin can actually start moving your arm, wrist, and hand, too. It is most certainly a weird and unwanted feeling. No doubt about it! Sometimes it will wake you up in the middle of the night, and you just can't possibly fall back asleep while having an itch you can't even scratch and having your hand curl up in different ways and forms. I have never experienced this feeling anywhere else on my body, but am certain others have.

I have come this far in this book without even mentioning the physical neuropathic pain more than 50% of people with this terrible disease experience every day, and every single night of their lives. I guess that's due to the simple fact that I don't really experience that particular type of pain too often. I happen to be very fortunate with that aspect of my MS, because I definitely wouldn't want to be forced to put up with that type of pain. It's very unfortunate for so many other MSers to have to deal with that pain all the time, almost non-stop.

But there is another type of pain many people with MS go through. This type of pain we experience is emotional. Sometimes we will laugh when things are sad, and cry when things are not sad at all. There are many times when we can't help shovel, mow the lawn, or even rake up the leaves that have fallen so gracefully off the cold branches of the trees. I know for a fact that this disturbs me a lot. It brings out that deep inner feeling of not being good enough to help out.

Another aspect of having MS that you very well may have to put up with is called Pseudobulbar Affect. This is the name of a strange phenomenon. It happens to be pretty common in people with this disease, and fortunately there is medicine to help treat it, so talk to your neurologist about this uncontrollable laughter and crying when you can.

Trust me, it's not a good feeling to laugh at something that's not funny, and to cry when something is supposed to be funny. Many people around you will quickly get the wrong idea about you, and that's understandable. I would look at myself as if I had two heads, too, if I didn't know and wasn't aware of the situation. This is definitely one of those symptoms many MSers and their caregivers have to put up with.

Something else that can be hard for some people to understand is the fact that I watch a movie I already saw before as if I've never seen it. I still laugh at funny parts and get sad at parts that are gloomy. Again, this seems to happen no matter how many times I have seen the show, or movie.

Another crazy experience for me with my MS is the feeling I get when I go into a hot tub, or jacuzzi. I start to feel pins and needles in my legs and I have to get out and cool off as quickly as possible. It starts to hurt me very quickly. Getting into hot water in a bath use to be a way doctors could tell if you had MS or not, because they would look at the symptoms it gave the person, or how it affected them after they got out. Obviously, this was well before the famous and much needed magnetic resonance imaging (MRI) machine. I wonder what type of machine they will come up with next. I am sure whatever it is will help doctors, patients, and loving caregivers even more, and that's what we all want.

Heat and humidity sure can bring on a lot of different terrible symptoms for us MSers. It's simply not good at all to have to feel that way. Even the cold weather makes my tremors worse and makes me move slower, both cognitively and physically. I start to shake like a little chiwawa. MS shows no mercy, or so it seems. I am currently shaking like crazy writing, or typing, this book. Patience sure is a wonderful virtue, and you are very fortunate if you happen to have it.

So with all of these different challenges life brings on at times, it is important to know that you have to keep your head up and move forward. You have to do what you have to do to get through what you have to get through. It may not be easy, but it's necessary. Keep moving forward, and try not to stay idle for too long of a time. Move what you are able to move with your body. It may take me a long time to do different tasks around the house, but at times, I am able to complete those tasks of such things as laundry and cleaning the dishes. Although there has been many times when I miss a spot or two on a plate or bowl. heck, sometimes a cup, as well. However, at least I am moving and getting some things done around the house. I am even able to sweep and mop some days when my energy level seems to be alright for the time being.

    At times, things happen so quickly. I remember being fearful that if I continue to get worse, then I wouldn't be able to hold my wife's hand while walking through the mall and while walking outside on the sidewalk, or anywhere else for that matter.

Well, wouldn't you know with the way MS works, I did happen to get worse and was unable to walk hand in hand with the very person I love and married years ago. It's a miracle and a half that she's still with me. I find it so sad knowing how much we take for granted without even being aware of it. Who would've thought I would eventually be so ill that I wouldn't be able to do something so simple, or something I use to do all the time? I surely didn't see it coming, and not many people would. I can't even put a necklace around her beautiful neck due to my tremors being so bad.

Speaking of crazy times with a crazy disease, there have been a few of these times that have fearfully occurred in the water. One crazy time was in the Atlantic Ocean. I thought I would be ok at first, but the strong and powerful waves proved otherwise. My leg muscles were just too weak and my balance was already shot. I didn't stand a chance much longer in the water with the waves, so I was fortunate enough to get out while I had the chance.

Another close call for me was in a lake years later. I figured there were no big and powerful waves and I would be safe out there with my two sons. Well, wouldn't you know that I ended up going too far out and my youngest son had to literally pull my hand until my head was out of the water. I don't think I'll ever forget that moment, nor would I want to. Why I just didn't swim is beyond my recollection, and many others, as well. Maybe it was shock. I was just unable to think straight. Such a great thing my son was next to me and knew exactly what to do. Thank God for those quick instincts that he had, because it literally saved my life.

The third and hopefully last time I came close to drowning is when I ended up falling out of a yellow and narrow kayak near the shoreline of a lake. It's such a good thing that I was strong enough to lift myself up after I fell right out of that yellow kayak in shallow water. It's another great thing that my wife and the lifeguard were close by helping me get and stay upright and steady.

The MS craziness doesn't even come close to stopping there. If I ever got the slightest low-grade fever, then I would easily become so stiff in my legs that it would lead to paralysis below my waist line. Wouldn't you know that I would have to go to the bathroom in this particular time that I was unable to be mobile, too. I absolutely hate having a fever and feeling sick, for so many different reasons, but at the same time can't always avoid it.

Sinus infections would always lead to this problem. So now I was totally congested in my nasal passages and head, and I got a fever on top of that. Let me tell you something you may already know. It's pretty hard blowing your nose when you have tremors and a fever. Good thing my wife makes sure that we always have plenty of Tylenol and Motrin on hand, just in case I should spike a fever out of the blue one day. This has helped me so many times. I am so grateful to have a wife who knows how to take care of me if and when needed. Trust me, I hate putting her in that situation. There have actually been times when our family had to help out, as well. Again, so grateful.

So I would like to throw something out there for you readers. For me, I usually use a tablespoon of honey with a tablespoon of apple cider vinegar whenever I start getting stuffy. This remedy appears to work well for me and helps prevent yet another sinus infection. You can even take it twice during the day, if you have to. Unfortunately though, it doesn't work well for everyone, and sometimes not even me, but I hope it works well for you if you try it. It's better than not trying anything at all.

I have also received bee pellets that have pollen in it that the bees collect and drop off in their hive. My cousin, who is also a nurse, knows that I get bad allergies that lead to a sinus infection most of the time, so she figured my body would form antibodies from these pollen filled pellets and prevent me from reacting to a lot of different allergens. I want to say that it seems to be working so far, and we are almost in June.

With all these many different challenges we have to face in life, we should remember that it could always be worse, because some people are actually diagnosed with a much more aggressive and terminal type of MS called Marburg's Variant MS. Let's always try to do the best we can in life, while we have it.

MY DIAGNOSIS

There were many different weird and strange things happening to me that I brushed off, but fortunately my wife thought it would be a good idea to go to the family doctor and get checked out and examined.

To begin with, just about every month like clockwork, I would feel dizzy and end up getting sick. However, this type of dizziness was different to me, because the room would feel like it was moving and shaking even with my eyes closed.

What a terrible feeling! I had no idea what caused it, and wasn't sure how to fix it, or prevent it from happening again. I would feel fine before bed, but would end up feeling like everything was shaking as I became awake lying on the bed later on with my eyes closed.

Something else happened, too. When I played full court basketball, I would end up tripping over my own feet after running up and down the court a couple times. I would also sweat a lot. I just figured I was out of shape, because I haven't exercised like that in a while, and my body just wasn't use to the strenuous workout on a warm and sunny day.

Yet another problem arose when I was in the house and I started walking into the walls, due to my lack of balance. I really felt as though I had to hold on to something, or I would easily fall down and hug the floor.

And the anomalies didn't stop there, either. I started to notice my hands shaking a lot and difficulty keeping my arms up and out in front of me for a while. It just felt as though my arms were too heavy and needed to rest. I again figured I was just out of shape and that it was normal to feel that way with me getting older and all.

I remember going to an ophthalmologist when I was younger, because when I looked at the pac-man screen with just my left eye open, I noticed extra dots on the TV screen. After that, I noticed that things looked a bit blurry when viewing them with just my left eye. I just figured I would need glasses to correct the blurriness and vision. No big deal!

So I ended up going to an eye doctor at a place called Pearl Vision. Well, while doing some eye exams and trying different lenses, the doctor just told me that no matter what lense I put on, my left eye will still be blurry. There was just nothing the doctor could do to help me see clearly out of my left eye.

At seventeen years old at the time, I didn't think about asking him any questions as to WHY my left eye was always blurry and WHY no lenses could fix it. I was just basically happy to not need glasses and went on with my day. I figured whatever the issue was would just eventually heal itself.

If that were to happen these days, then I'm sure the ophthalmologist would tell me I have optic neuritis and that such a thing is common in people with multiple sclerosis. I am also pretty sure that I would even be recommended to see a neurologist.

Well, none of that happened, and I was alright with it, because as long as I view everything with both my eyes, then nothing is blurry and everything is alright.

It wasn't until about ten years later that I would be diagnosed with multiple sclerosis (MS).

This time, a neurologist was telling me to look at a colored piece of paper while covering my good eye and explain what I see. So after thinking about how I would describe the colored piece of paper in front of me, I finally decided to tell him that the color looked dull and plain. I didn't see what the big deal was, or the point of describing a specific color on a piece of paper that the doctor was holding in his hand.

After that description, the doctor told me to switch the eye I was looking out of to the other eye. With the same piece of paper in front of me, I just could not begin to fathom how bright the color actually was. It wasn't dull at all, but much rather a highlighted color. I was dumbfounded! It was as if it was a magic trick.

However, this was not even the first neurologist I saw. The first neurologist I saw told me to go home and have a couple beers to help with my tremors, and that nothing was wrong with me. This was after he supposedly looked at my MRI. How could this be? It really makes me wonder how that could of happened knowing what I know today.

Well, my wife and I decided to see a different neurologist after that, and sure enough, this neurologist looked at the same MRI scan, and showed me the multiple lesions that I had on my brain and diagnosed me with multiple sclerosis.

Ok, so now we have a name that describes the type of problems and anomalies I have been having and experiencing in my life. Next, my wife and I have to go home and figure out what type of a disease modifying therapy to start after reading all of the material about the different medications and possible adverse reactions.

This already felt weird, because usually you see a doctor and a certain medication is prescribed for you in order to help you feel better. This was completely backwards. This time, the decision was in our hands to decide what treatment I should start taking.

Another weird feeling is the fact that I was preventing my MS from getting any worse, but not feeling better within a few days like I just started an antibiotic prescribed to me by my family doctor. This way of doing things for my health was completely awkward.

I guess MS can be a bit confusing for doctors, too. I didn't really think that was possible at the time. Boy, have I learned a lot about not only having a disease, but how confusing it can be for so many people. Looks like I'm not the only one confused.

Next thing we had to do after the diagnosis was think about what we would do without me bringing home a regular paycheck all the time. We ended up deciding to apply for social security disability (SSD) and my amazing wife would now be the breadwinner of the house. Meanwhile, after months went by, I ended up getting approved for SSD. All the forms we had to fill out and complete a particular way helped move the process along. I even called the person in charge of my case about different medications I started while waiting for the approval or the denial. I felt like I had to do something to help with my case.

TREMORS

Through the years with this horrible and debilitating disease, I began having awful tremors with both of my hands in the hot and cold weather. I could no longer write legibly. The words were basically just scribble. Once the pen touched the paper, pen marks would just quickly go all over the place. I would have no control whatsoever, and the pen would go anywhere and everywhere. I actually remember one episode happening to me back in the seventh grade. Fortunately, that went away the next day at school, but now the only thing I could do these days is sign my name, because that didn't have to be written neatly. Good thing!

There have been many times when I couldn't zipper my coat or even button my shirt. This can be very frustrating. My hands would just go everywhere uncontrollably. Boy, those days when I could do it easily seemed to have been taken for granted by me. Who would have known that one day you wouldn't be able to do such simple tasks? It makes me wonder what endeavors I can do these days that I might not be able to do further on in the future. I guess only time will tell. Let's hope there's no more stubborn progression of this disease.

Another lesson I learned about having tremors is that you have to figure out what hand happens to shake more than the other, so that you don't try carrying anything with it. Just take it slow and be careful, especially if you are going from one room to another. Tremors have forced me to use two hands when I shave, pick up a drink, brush my hair, and even brush my teeth. Again, many of us tend to take a lot of our abilities for granted. It often takes a disability to realize the ability you once had. It also takes a disability to see gifts that you have that you were not aware of and that were hidden. There's always a better way to look at things, so try to remember that and be as positive as you can possibly be.

After many months with this problem of my fine motor skills, I decided to start learning how to write with my left hand, due to the simple fact that it's not as shaky and a little more controllable at times. Well, it sure did feel weird writing with my left hand, but the words came out to be a lot more legible as long as I took my time. You would be amazed at the talented abilities you have within yourself the more you practice doing something your body isn't use to doing.

So now that I knew my left hand didn't shake as much as my dominant right hand, I started using my left hand to help bring the spoon and fork to my mouth with food. This ended up working better and being more successful than using my right hand that would shake so much. Trust me, the food would easily go all around the room and everywhere else, if I tried using my dominant right hand. In order for me to pick up my drink, I would need to use both hands. It just doesn't take much for liquid to go all over the place in a hurry. One uncontrollable tremor is more than enough and all you need to make and generate chaos.

After many months of having these tremors, I tried going on a medication to help calm the shaking down. Although my tremors did get a little better, I now had problems urinating. There were times when I would have to go to either the hospital or an urgent care to have a catheter put in me in order to release the urine from my bladder and void. Who would've thought you'd have difficulties doing something so natural? Not me!

Needless to say, I decided to stop the medication that helped treat my tremors. Shortly after doing so, I could urinate without a problem again. Interesting how that happened. Although, I should mention that those occurrences still happen for me, just not nearly as much. I also want to mention the fact that it is possible to get those little clumps in your urine if you consume too much protein.

Let me share another story about having popcorn at the movies. Well, when you have tremors, there is a very good chance that the popcorn does not end up in your mouth like you think it would, or planned. Sometimes it would end up on my shirt and roll to the chair I'm sitting on, and eventually fall to the floor. It must be hard to keep that movie theater clean after the movie with candy and popcorn all over the floor. Anyhow, I learned that it would be better to use my left hand to get popcorn or candy directly to my mouth. Fortunately, it works a lot better that way. The popcorn and candy actually make it all the way to my mouth without losing it to my shirt, or to the floor.

  Of course, and to find out the hard way that the same problem occurs when eating french fries or potato chips. Heck, it happens when you eat just about any type of snack, or food with your hands.

Ok, so I was doing some research one day about how weighted silverware helps people with tremors eat more smoothly and steadily. I just had to give that a try, and fortunately my wife bought me a set. It even came with a soup spoon. Long and behold, I was able to eat my food without it dropping off the fork and spoon, and flying across the room as if it had a jet propulsion connected to it and ready to defy gravity. Fortunately, I actually had more control with the eating utensil and food going from the plate to my mouth. What a blessing! I tell you, the things we take for granted are out of this world and downright amazing. We don't even realize it many times.

One of the things I still had problems with, though, was taking the shell off a hardboiled egg. What a disaster that was. I simply couldn't do it successfully. I admitted defeat. My hands would just go everywhere. Sometimes even the hard-boiled egg would get mushed or ruined while shells would go all over the place. It's not good when you add a mess you have to clean up when you are already feeling fatigued. With fatigue, the mess can be a lot bigger than it seems to be to the eye.

Another challenging moment in time is when my phone is on the nightstand and I attempt to pick it up when the phone rings. Either the phone would grow wings and fly across the room, or I would pick it up and accidentally hang up on the person. Good thing my family is so understanding, because they have been on the other end of the call plenty of times.

Moving along, who ever thought clipping your fingernails and toenails would be so hard and take up so much time. Well, when you have tremors and your legs are stiff as a board, you will certainly have a problem clipping your nails. It doesn't take a genius to figure that one out. Patience and perseverance are going to be your dearest friends for this job. Hopefully, these friends are by your side, because you will need them, especially if it's hot and humid. I just can't seem to quantify the effect of humidity and heat. It's a downright nightmare, and most of you MSers sadly know this already.

DOING THINGS DIFFERENTLY

Creativity and cleverness sure do come in handy with multiple sclerosis (MS), and you are blessed the moment you have them, especially with all the brain fog and fatigue you experience throughout the day.

There are so many different tough lessons someone has to learn with MS. The sooner you happen to learn them, the better. I have learned that instead of making a complete journey from the kitchen sink to the oven with a pot of water, I must first put the pot down on a chair or stool along the way, and reposition myself before bringing the pot of water over to the stove from the stool. This way I don't end up spilling the water in the pot with my tremors. Remember, knowledge is power and what you don't know may end up hurting you. If you end up spilling boiling water all over the place, then you will most likely get burned and hurt yourself, or even hurt the people around you at the time, as well. Who wants to do that? Surely not me!

    After the food has boiled long enough, I have to make sure I put a hotplate on the stool before I put the pot on it, then reposition myself before I pick the pot up again and put the contents in the strainer I already put in the sink. This procedure ends up being more with these extra steps, but that's how I beat adversity and get the job done safely. The job may even take a lot of extra steps at times, but again, better safe than sorry. Sometimes taking that extra step makes a world of difference. I feel as though it's also important to ask for help if you need to. Try not to be bashful, because people are usually happy to help you in any way that they can.

    I have also learned to make sure I put my hot drink in a large mug so I don't end up spilling it all over myself or someone else along my journey to the table, or wherever else I may be going. In fact, if it has a lid on the cup, then it's even safer and smarter. With the tremors I mentioned in chapter 3, carrying anything anywhere successfully, can surely be a challenge, simply due to the fact that you have no idea when a big tremor is going to occur and you accidentally throw a plate or cup somewhere across the room simply by accident.

It is also a good idea to see an occupational therapist (OT) to help you have a better day in the life of a person with multiple sclerosis. Seeing an occupational therapist can help you see other ways to get things done around the house. You can really learn how to conserve your energy in many different ways, and we all know how important that is. Especially when you wake up fatigued and carry it with you throughout the entire day like a heavy coat that you just can't take off.

Another important thing to remember is the fact that you should wear socks that have grip on the bottom. This way you can get up easier from the couch or chair without your feet slipping. This is also very important when you have to use the bathroom, because you are able to get up quicker. Every moment counts when you have urgency and frequency. You simply can't afford the time it takes slipping on the floor and repositioning your stiff legs and feet when you suddenly get the urge to use the restroom. You really want to try to make everything as simple as you possibly can. If this means wearing socks with grips at the end, then that is what is necessary for you to do. If you feel like you have to explain yourself, then simply say you would really like to make it to the bathroom before you end up going in your clothes.

By the way, being fatigued all the time and having tremors makes simple things a lot harder to accomplish. If you don't make it to the bathroom on time, then that means you are going to have to clean yourself up and clean up the area. Taking a shower is already taxing enough on a regular day for people with MS, but now you may have to clean yourself up for the second time in the day.

SHAME AND DEPENDENCE

When the time comes when someone else has to put on your shoes and tie them for you, then it is very common and understandable that you start to feel shameful and more dependent, because you can't do it yourself, and now someone else has to do something for you that was at one time such an easy task for you to do yourself. Although it is always wonderful to have the help and assistance from someone, you just feel awful and wish you could do it yourself like you were more accustomed to doing before this terrible disease took control of your body and started tearing apart your myelin sheath like Pac-Man eating the dots on the board. Before your legs became so stiff that it became difficult and challenging to bend your own legs and simply raise them up. Before your life added about thirty or forty years to your age just like that. As if getting older wasn't already a tough task to handle by itself, but now you have to face it earlier in life and somehow do the best you can to deal with it.

    Another example of needing someone's help is when you have fallen and literally can't get up on your own. No matter how long and how much you try to do it yourself. You almost feel like a beetle stuck on its back moving all of its legs just trying to turn over and get up, but can't. With MS, this appears to be very common to be down and not able to get up on your own. You just don't seem to have the necessary strength, balance, and flexibility to move your own legs and feet the way you need to in order to simply get up and be stable enough to stand on your own. Sometimes it's even hard getting help up, or back on your feet from the floor from the chair you're sitting on, or even your wheelchair, because you just can't bend your stiff legs, or you don't have good enough flexibility at that particular time of the day. The statement about "losing it if you don't use it" sure is true in many cases, especially if you should happen to have MS. What can you do about it when you have to depend on a wheelchair and a cane to get around, though? The answer is exercise as much as you can and try not to have your muscles stiffen up and get weak. It is a big challenge, and much easier said than done. Feel free to also talk to your neurologist about any of the challenges that you are currently experiencing. Keep moving is a wonderful saying and logo in different MS magazines and certain places, but with stiffness and fatigue, it especially doesn't mean it's going to be easy, but it sure is necessary.

There even comes the time when you have to depend on someone helping you get out of the car and become more stable on your feet after you finally stand up. Let's not forget all the help you need to get in the car, as well. Sometimes your stiff legs just don't want to bend at the knee, so someone needs to help bend them for you as you attempt to sit down in the car. This is very true especially on hot and humid days. There are also times when you need help lifting your leg up high enough to get in the car or truck in the first place. If it happens to be a truck without the foot bar, then you may very well need to step up on a portable stepping stool before you can even try to get in safely. Many of us MSers just don't seem to have the ability to lift our legs up that high. For those of you that can, please try your best not to lose it by keeping flexible and strong. Unfortunately, it is still possible that this disease progresses and makes your symptoms even worse over time. Exercise as much as you yourself can do, though. For me in particular, there is a very fine line that falls between doing too much and not doing enough, or at least feeling that I am not doing enough.

When it comes time to eat, I would usually need help carrying whatever I have to the table, if I don't want any of it to drop down on the floor and make a huge and much unwanted mess. Heck, I remember trying to carry two bowls of mint chocolate chip ice cream from the kitchen to the dining room table at one time. I thought I was doing alright, but next thing I knew, I ended up shaking and dropping both bowls of ice cream on the off-white tiles on the kitchen floor. All that soon to be eaten delicious looking ice cream for me and my son ended up all over the kitchen floor. What felt like a great idea for me at the time just ended up not to be my smartest one. That's been known to happen at times. I would have to say that asking for help carrying the two bowls of ice cream sure would have been a great idea.

      Talking about being dependent, one of the toughest and most challenging moments for people with MS is when they have the slightest type of fever. Being sensitive to any type of heat, in general, when the body decides to do something like ward off an infection of some sort and raise its own body temperature, it gets to a point where moving at all is extremely challenging. This is when you know it's time for tylenol, ibuprofen, and very possibly an antibiotic. What a big difference that medication can do for you. It's like night and day. The sooner you can start the medication, then the better for you and your caregiver. that helps the body cool off and lower the inflammation of your multiple scars in your brain and spinal cord, is a good thing, as long as you go about it in a safe way. For instance, do NOT put yourself in an ice cold bath tub to help lower your body temperature. Instead of going to such extreme measures, get a cool washcloth to put over your head. The safer, the better, because it doesn't seem to take too much to need help for an individual with MS. A lot of things can happen in a very small amount of time.

We have to try to stay as healthy as we can. If anything little happens to us, then we may very well need to be more dependent, and that is by far not my goal in life.

I remember needing to go to the hospital one night via ambulance, and the emergency room physician was so amazed when my fever broke and how I looked and felt immediately afterwards. You go from being stiff as a board and still, to being able to talk more and move around. It's truly amazing! I was a total different person after my fever broke. I would imagine I looked a lot different, too.

I don't want to forget to mention the sad feeling I get whenever the driveway needs to be shoveled or snowblowed and the time a car gets stuck, but you just can't help like you use to be able to. You can't shovel and you can't help push the car out, but you sure can help yourself and the people around you by NOT trying to do too much and end up getting hurt. All you can do is watch. Talk about feeling shameful and dependent.

NEEDING A WHEELCHAIR

Being that wheelchair use is in the deck of cards I have to play with in my life, I am able to see certain anomalies that many people wouldn't think of on a usual and casual day. It just wouldn't even cross their mind. Some of these problems and hardships occur to me when I am in a wheelchair and the kind person pushing me is trying to get around obstacles such as a curb, or even stairs if they don't have a ramp where you're going. I know this may seem very small for many people, but it's rather big for an individual in a wheelchair, and the person pushing you in the wheelchair, as well. Some restaurants are not even wheelchair accessible. The fact that I'm being pushed in the wheelchair simply means that I am not the only one concerned about these crazy and unwanted obstacles. There are about 400,000 people with MS alone in the United States of America. This doesn't even count for people with other challenges in life that need to use a wheelchair. Let's not forget our veterans that may need to use a wheelchair after battling in war, or just growing old.

Instead of going five to fifteen feet in order to get in a particular place, we now have to go forty or more feet. Even many fast food restaurants are not easily accessible by people in a wheelchair. It's just another one of those things people don't realize until they have to use a wheelchair themselves or push a wheelchair with someone in it.

There was this one popular restaurant that happened to have steps in order to reach the next level of seating, and at the time, it was very busy, and getting to the next level was a must, or we wouldn't be eating any food from there inside sitting comfortably at a table. Well, yet again, my wonderful wife and our great children helped to lift me in the wheelchair so that we could all sit at a table together at Pizza Hut. You really want that food once you start smelling their Pizza and everything else they cook in the kitchen. You would think there would be a ramp for someone in a wheelchair, but sadly there wasn't. The things we have to do for pizza hut pizza can surely be excessive and challenging when the people that you are with have to lift the wheelchair you are in up to the next level. As if you didn't already feel bad enough needing to use a wheelchair in the first place.

Yet another problem is going to the beach. Just try to push someone in a wheelchair through the sand, or try to bring your motorized scooter on the beach through the sand. I am very sure it will be extremely hard to do, if not impossible.

Some beaches do have a way for someone using a wheelchair to get closer to the water, though. I always feel good about that. It helps me and my caregiver a lot. Just because I am too afraid to get in the water on a hot and humid day doesn't mean everyone I'm with is, too.

Another good idea many people have when it comes to needing to use a wheelchair is putting a sidewalk not too far from the lake. I can definitely understand not putting a sidewalk close to an ocean, though. That would be a bit too risky with tides coming in during the day. Someone using a wheelchair on a sidewalk too close to the ocean in this circumstance, is in a lot of danger.

Talking about different places when using a wheelchair can be difficult to maneuver, moving a wheelchair is extremely hard to do around certain parks. These places can be very challenging if they are not wheelchair accessible. Moving a wheelchair around in gravel and wood chips can obviously be very challenging. It's not like we are ready to play at the park, but maybe our children are. With the way things are happening in the world these days, being closer to your children may be a good idea at times.

FATIGUE

Ok, so what exactly is fatigue? Don't we all experience moments of feeling tired? Well, we all get tired, but not everyone feels like you can't do anything because you're too exhausted to move most of the time and feel like collapsing to the floor because your legs feel so weak and you have no energy at all. Sometimes you can feel overly tired when you are just sitting down on the couch or somewhere else in or around the house on a chair or on anything you can possibly find to sit on.

Try and picture yourself just sleeping most of the day and all night long mostly every day. This involves taking a number of naps a day, and still feeling like you don't have the energy to accomplish much at all. With all of this sleeping every day, you still have a difficult time thinking, or focusing, because your very own brain is in a fog. Even simple things become hard to think about. You just feel so tired that you want to close your eyes and take a nap no matter what time of the day it is.

And these don't have to all be naps on your bed, but also places like the couch and in the car on your way to go somewhere. You're just feeling as though you're not in the game, so to speak.

Heck, I remember driving to different places and finding myself actually opening my eyes while driving, because for the life of me, I just could not keep my eyes open. That was scary!

Fatigue is also when you go to sleep instead of helping put the groceries away after shopping. It's not that you don't want to help, but more like you are exhausted and feel like you're going to collapse to the floor if you stand any longer. You are out of the strength you need to stay on your feet and to stay awake and alert.

Fatigue is staying home and sleeping, because you don't have the energy to go out with your family and be active with them. I can't even imagine everything I missed during all the years of having and dealing with MS and its many symptoms.

When you feel as exhausted as you do throughout most of the day everyday, you start thinking of ways to minimize your activity level, in hopes that it'll help you feel less tired. There were many times when the dishes would just pile up until someone could help me clean them. A lot of times, I would just rinse the spoon I used to stir my coffee and reuse my cup that I just rinsed out. I wanted to conserve as much energy as I could, and small things add up quickly.

There were also many times when the dirty laundry would keep piling up until someone was able to help me clean the clothes and towels during their own busy day.

Let's not forget the times I didn't even have the strength and energy to stand on my very own feet to take a shower. You know you're experiencing fatigue when you can't even do that. Even shaving seemed to take a lot of energy out of me. It would feel as though I would have to take another nap afterwards.

Fatigue means you can only help out a little bit with the chores around the house. Sometimes I would use one day just to sweep and the following day to mop. Some other days would be spent trying to take care of the laundry, or the dishes. There are simply so many different missions to try and complete just inside the house, and you may have to break the big missions down to size a bit when going through fatigue. This is important to remember.

Another important idea to put in your head somewhere is the fact that you can do many different jobs in the house little by little. There are many different examples of making a big project smaller. The first example will deal with dishes. Having fatigue during the day is tough, so instead of cleaning twenty dirty dishes at once, you can start with cleaning about five awful looking dishes, and save the rest for later on during the day. This way you at least started cleaning the plates, bowls, pans, pots, and silverware.

Secondly, rather than starting about three loads of laundry one right after the other, you can rather start off with one load and do another load later on in the day. You may very well need help, so if the laundry has to wait, then it may very well have to wait until some can help you.

Thirdly, instead of dusting the entire house from one room to the next without taking a break, dust a particular room like the living room and take a break before you start dusting the dining room. Breaks are important to take, especially when you are experiencing fatigue.

Just try to remember that when you are sadly dealing with fatigue, you may very likely need some help from someone, and I think it is important to break down big projects to smaller projects and do a little at a time. It may not be a good idea for anyone to paint the whole house at once, but much rather compartmentalizing and doing one part at a time. When building a staircase, you don't make all the stairs at once, but much rather one step at a time. It's also like a tall building needing to be built one level at a time. Even the Great Wall of China that can be seen from the Moon was not built in one day. This is how big projects are made smaller.

    It is such a blessing that I have family members to help me out. They do as much as they can to help me when they see that I'm tired and falling asleep throughout the day. Therefore, it can be pretty easy to assume a person with MS experiencing a high level of fatigue most of the time day after day, is just being lazy, but I assure you, that is not the case. Laziness and fatigue are two different problems that can easily be construed as one.

Laziness is when you have the energy to complete a task, but just don't want to, or care to. Whereas fatigue is when you desperately want to complete a task, but there is absolutely not enough energy in your body to do so. Trust me, if someone is experiencing fatigue, then even the simplest endeavor such as changing your very own shirt, is downright difficult to do. It will be hard to even start lifting your own arms up. I truly have to say that feeling beyond exhausted all the time is terrible. It is most certainly not a high quality of life.

Let's also remember that simply walking on a dry sidewalk can seem as though a person with MS is walking through inches of mud. Not only can it be hard to keep your balance, but walking a short distance like a city block, can feel like walking a mile. That can be one very good reason why people with multiple sclerosis feel as though they have to stop walking and take a much needed break.

COGNITIVE

So how does multiple sclerosis (MS) affect the way you think? Well, for me, I believe this is twofold, or even more. In one sense, I was able to go back to college and graduate with a degree, but in the other sense, it took a lot of time studying. And I mean a lot.

There were many times when I had to study material I had already studied, because the information I was learning felt like I never read it before, even though I have not only read it before, but I have also sat at the table and already studied it, as well. I just wasn't able to retain information quickly, such as only reading the material once and you understand the information good enough to take a test, and do well. That's just not me. My mind works differently.

No, I had to read the material a good number of times for it to be retained in my mind, or sink in. Especially when it came time to learn different types of math. In so many instances, the road may be hard and challenging, but achieving your goal is paramount and life changing, no matter how long it may take you, so try not to give up on your dreams and aspirations, and know there may be a good chance of everything coming together for you with hard work and perseverance. Don't just give up and take the easy way out.

Heat and humidity wouldn't help matters in the cognitive department at all when it came time for studying, either. That would just prolong the time needed to understand something even more. The heat and humidity would put me in a brain fog. This is where nobody ever wants to be. It's something like knowing the song you're listening to, but just can't recall the name of the band that sings it, even though you know you know it and it's just at the tip of your tongue. It's just so frustrating to be that close to recalling something, but unable to for the life of you.

Another example of going through a moment of brain fog is when you look at someone as if that person has two heads, because you can't understand what is being said at all. The conversation he/she just had with you feels as if a different language was being spoken, a language you definitely don't know and are unaware of. Being in a brain fog makes understanding simple things hard, and more challenging, because you just don't get it. Your brows easily go down as though you're thinking very hard, but are sadly confused nonetheless.

I actually use to help tutor math and help out with homework, but I would have to first spend a lot of time reading the material and figuring it out to the best of my ability. In the meantime, the person I was helping needed to wait, and it usually took a lot of time. I am very fortunate the people I helped had patience and were very nice, because we all needed it.

    After reading many MS magazines, I learned that some of the things that may help you think more sharply and activate your brain are different mind games such as chess and Sudoku. These are just two of the many different mind games that may help you stay out of brain fog. Luminosity is another brain game along with brain age 1 and brain age 2. I was fortunate enough to get both of these brain age games from my wife that can be used on the Nintendo DS. It's also important to stick with the brain game, because you can actually get better over time.

Another activity that helps me turn the wheels upstairs in my mind, is reading a book, or reading articles that interest me in a magazine or newspaper. It just seems to help me think better and focus more at times. We all know that every single day is different, however.

Another interesting way to get your mind going is simply getting in a routine to think about what you had to eat last night. If this is too simple for you, then try and think what you had for dinner two nights ago, and even three nights ago. Try to do this on a regular basis and see how far back you can go. If you master that exercise, then include what you had for breakfast and lunch, as well.

If this seems to bore you, because it's so easy, then you can even try adding what you had to drink at each meal. This will definitely make it more challenging for you.

I feel as though the mind is like technology in a way, because if it's working well then it's great, but if it's not working well, then it can be very frustrating and aggravating, to say the least.

There are some days that go by when I am forgetful. I forget to bring the car keys to the car. So I get all the way there to the car, but then have to go back in the house to get the keys. There have been other times when I get to the car and realize I forgot my phone, but remembered the keys. Sometimes I have my car keys and phone and get to the store, just to realize that I forgot my wallet when I'm about to pay for everything I already put on the counter next to the register. Good thing this doesn't always happen though.

IDENTITY

So who are you now? For many of us with multiple sclerosis (MS), life as we once knew it, changes drastically and quickly. You can go from working 72 hour weeks to zero hours a week, in a blink of an eye. You can also go from making multiple errands to not being able to make as many errands anymore.

For me, an MS warrior not decided by choice, does all I can to roll with the punches that life appears to throw my way, especially the surprise uppercut that you never saw coming, or a surprise southpaw hit to your head that you didn't think was coming at all.

Car maintenance is another thing that changes as your stubborn MS progresses and makes you become even more disabled. Believe it or not, I use to change my own oil and oil filter when it came time to. I even added transmission fluid, or transaxle fluid when it needed it. However, now it has changed to us needing to go somewhere and pay to get it done. I have become a dependent person that relies more and more on other people, instead of an independent person that use to do many different types of tasks myself, including work hard for a living.

The roles in the relationship have changed from you going out to work and bringing home most of the income and providing health insurance for the family to her working a lot more and bringing home most of the income and providing health insurance for the family. Your new job now is trying to help out more with household chores such as laundry, dishes, cooking and baking, sweeping, mopping, and a bunch of other tasks. So yes, this part of your identity has changed. You have a different role now, but so does your wife.

Without a doubt, you seem to lose a big part of yourself with this crazy illness. I mean really, you're simply not the same person as you once were before this terrible disease invaded your body in so many ways. You can't be that gentleman you use to be if you can't even open the door for your wonderful wife and can't slide the chair back and in for her at the table. You can't hold her hand as you walk around the mall and different stores either. It would help if she didn't need to push you in a wheelchair and you didn't have to walk at a slow pace using a cane. Surely, having good mobility would be a great help, but that doesn't seem to be in the deck of cards that were handed me, so I have to think of other ways to be a gentleman.

    Good thing you can still be a nice and thoughtful gentleman in other ways. You can still have flowers and a card sent her way, or a cup of coffee if you happen to both be out together, or you happen to be able to surprise her at work with one. A box of chocolate is another good idea at times, as long as she is not allergic. Let's not forget some movie tickets once in a while, and even to suggest she goes out with her girlfriends for dinner or shopping. That can make her feel good and gives her a little break from the everyday hasle.

Being that you're not the person with wonderful abilities to do many different things like before you became so ill, let's hope the person you have been forced to become with this awful disease is still thoughtful and nice, especially with many swift changes to the role you use to have in the relationship. Let's not forget that her role has also changed, though. In fact, she may have to work multiple jobs now that you're not bringing home a weekly, or biweekly paycheck.

So yes, not only has your very own identity changed, but her identity has also been forced to change, as well. You may not be the same person you were before, but you may still be a good person. Although you may experience fatigue, your values and morals are still ingrained in you. You still know right from wrong. You still know how to be a nice and caring person. That part of you is still within yourself, and hopefully has not changed at all. Hopefully!

MEDICATIONS

Ok, so having MS for many people means a life of trying different medications, or different disease modifying therapies, because we generally listen to the suggestions our neurologist has that we have to visit at least twice a year. We want to be in the best possible shape we can be in, considering our circumstance. We are told that we should go on a type of medicine, or therapy that will slow down the stubborn progression of multiple sclerosis (MS). As we well know, if the terrible disease progresses and gets worse, then we are most likely going to be more disabled, and not be able to do as much as we were able to do before, at least not as easily and quickly. The things we miss when we no longer have them is tough. Some days more than others, but what else can we do but try our best and keep moving forward and onward with our life.

By the way, don't be afraid to change your neurologist if you feel as though you have to and need to. I have read many stories where people were not happy with the neurologist they were seeing. Even I have needed to change neurologists twice in my life so far. Sometimes you just have to. When a neurologist tells you to go home and have a couple beers to help with your tremors, then you know something is wrong and that you need to see a different neurologist. That is like a dead giveaway. Sad but true.

Viewing graphs can help us better understand the difference between how life was for people with MS before having disease modifying therapies, and how living with this awful disabling disease is now that we have a good number of medications to help with so many different types of people living life in the slow lane. These different medications are taken either by injections, infusions, or even oral pills these days. The many different medications that are now available to help people with MS have come a long way, but there still isn't a cure. Hopefully, there will be a cure very soon. I have heard and read that maybe there will be a cure five to ten years from now, but who knows for sure. This cure may come sooner and it may come later than five to ten years.

However, before we had multiple medications to help slow down the inevitable progression and disability of MS, people generally got worse even quicker than they do today, because we have medications to help fight the progression of MS these days. Obviously, this means MSers became even more and more disabled at a faster pace beforehand. So let's remember to be thankful for these advancements in medicine these days, because it could mean a higher quality of life for many. In turn, a better life for not only the person with MS, but also the people around them and the caregivers, as well.

While managing to live with this frightful and frustrating disease, you learn so much, if you are open to such knowledge and willing to learn more. I know from experience that it can be very tough to learn while being in a brain fog all the time, but even if you have to read something over and over again to have it stick in your head, then it very well might be important to know and to try to remember, and thus worthwhile for you.

Technology has come a long way, and we should embrace it and learn how to use it if we can. I know I often put reminders on my phone, and it's a very good thing I do, because this way I can actually remember to do something I'm supposed to when that alarm goes off, such as go to an appointment, or ask someone to bring the garbage and recyclable bins outside by the curb to be picked up the following morning. These reminders also help me remember to pay certain bills when they are due, instead of facing a termination. In matter of fact, many people ask me to put a reminder on my phone for them, too. I am more than happy to help in any way I can, so I definitely don't mind doing that. There comes a time for everyone when we simply forget something. We have all been down that path before.

Something else that I know is that with fatigue, it is often hard and challenging not to fall asleep while reading a book, or anything else for that matter. It seems as though the eyelids get super heavy, and impossible to keep open. Especially on hot and humid days. Heck, even rainy days don't help with that situation. Fatigue is downright tough and cruel. No doubt about it, and no need to sugar coat it.

So in my lifetime, after being diagnosed with MS, I have tried some different disease modifying therapies to help me feel well. I also wanted, and hoped, that I could halt my MS progression and reverse the damage that has already taken place. One of the many things I learned with this tricky and debilitating disease, is that even if you happen to feel well, or as well as you possibly can at the time, you may still be going through a progression of this disease. Thus the reason why I say it's tricky. Just when you think one thing about MS, it's another, or when you think you're doing well, it ends up being that you have become worse.

Anyhow, I have tried medications such as Copaxone, Novantrone, Ampyra, Tysabri, Gilenya, and now low dose naltrexone (LDN). Personally, I feel as though adding LDN to my other two medications is the best idea for me ever, because I feel the best when I am taking all three of the medications. You can read more about this in the following chapter, but in the meantime, I feel as though it is important to know that going without Ampyra for me wasn't good at all. It appears as though LDN is a great addition to the MS therapy we are already taking. It makes me feel as though I have a better quality of life when I take LDN. It also makes me feel as though I have three pieces of the puzzle out of four, instead of just one or two pieces. Maybe one day there will be another MS therapy medication that will put all of the pieces together for us. We will feel completely whole again.

As many of us MSers, I started on copaxone thirteen years ago in 2004. My wife and I both thought it was a good idea, as well. I mean after going through all the options and reading material the neurologist sent home with us, copaxone sounded like the best option for us. It sure felt different deciding what medication I was going to go on. I was totally use to the doctor doing that for me, but this time, it was up to me and my wife.

    I didn't like needles to begin with, but rotating to all the different sites wasn't actually bad, until it came time to do my abdomen region. This area was bad for me, because I didn't like bringing the needle to myself in that particular region. I remember that it took me a little longer than an hour trying to stick myself in the abdomen with a needle. I thought for sure I was going to do it and came so close, but then I had to get psychologically pumped up just to try it again. I came so close so many times, but my mind seemed to of stopped me from going all the way and doing it. It feels as though my mind was pushing my hand away. It was a tough and very challenging moment in my life, and I finally proceeded to stick myself with a needle subcutaneously in my stomach area. Insane! That was such a big obstacle to overcome for me.

I tell you, it sure was a blessing when they came out with the autoject pen. What a lifesaver! I didn't have to see the needle after I loaded it in the special compartment. After looking and directing, all I had to do was press a button to give myself a shot. I didn't have any more problems after using that very innovative invention.

Well about a year later, my MS continued to progress, and my walking ability just became worse and worse. The progression of my disease made me and my wife question if I should change to a more aggressive neurologist. After finding out another neurologist is prescribing a stronger type of medicine in which could help me walk better, I switched. I just figured I wasn't going to sit around when the option of getting better was right there in front of me. How could I? Why should I?

This switch led to me being prescribed my second type of medication to help treat multiple sclerosis, novantrone. I still took my daily copaxone shot, but this time, I would also take a type of chemotherapy by IV. I heard some good things about this medicine, so I was hopeful and excited to try it. My wife and I are looking for a good change and we're eager to see improvements.

Well, after I received my first infusion, my wife took me home, and I slept on and off for an entire week. I never felt as tired and exhausted before in my entire life.

After I finally started to wake up and regain my strength, I went outside and noticed I didn't need my cane any more. I actually remember running and racing my cousin on foot in the backyard. Things were looking real good for me and the future appeared to be bright. So many good ideas were running through my mind. If I continue to improve, then I should be able to go back to work and bring home health insurance for the family and a good paycheck.

However, due to the fact that this type of medicine can weaken your heart muscles if used more than eight times in your life, my wife and I decided I would stop taking it after my second and third infusion, because I wasn't getting the same positive results anymore, anyway. In fact, I started to need my cane again. I was sliding back to where I was before my first infusion. Just when I thought things were looking good and that I made the right decision about what medicine to take. I guess not! The future started to look a bit on the dark side again, or at least a little less hopeful and promising with treating this disease. I really didn't think I would be able to go back to work now.

My neurologist decided to have me do a trial on ampyra while remaining on copaxone. I couldn't believe how much energy I started to have with this new medication. I was actually able to do more dishes during the day, and my fatigue level went down a bit. The speed of my walking also increased. This was good news. I have been on ampyra ever since I started it many years ago. By the way, it helps that the pharmaceutical company has a great program and helps pay for this walking pill. Long and behold, ampyra also helps with balance. Another common anomaly people with MS have.

As time kept passing by and moving forward, it was recommended I try a different approach of battling my MS, so I stopped taking my daily shots of copaxone, and started to have a monthly infusion of Tysabri (natalizumab). I was on this Tysabri for about a year before my neurologist decided to have my blood tested for the John Cunningham virus (JC virus, or JCV). It is believed that if you test positive for this JC virus while on Tysabri, then the chance of getting progressive multifocal leukoencephalopathy (PML) increases. This rare viral disease can be fatal. Especially without a cure for PML.

    I did end up testing positive for the JC virus antibody, so to decrease my chance of getting PML, it was recommended I stop taking my monthly infusions of Tysabri.

Sure enough, I ended up stopping Tysabri and going on a different disease-modifying therapy (DMT) called Gilenya (fingolimod). With the first time taking this pill, you have to be at a Gilenya medical site, or facility, a doctor's office, or even at home with the Gilenya home program. This is necessary so they can monitor your heart on an electrocardiogram for six hours and make sure nothing drastic changes, such as a slower heart rate. You also had to stay so they can do some blood work on you and run tests.

When starting gilenya, it is also important to see a good eye doctor for an eye exam. It is possible to get what is called macular edema, so you are tested by an ophthalmologist after being on

Gilenya. The doctors want to see what your baseline is, so it's easier to see if there are any negative changes after taking Gilenya.

While still being on Gilenya for years, I have also started taking low dose naltrexone (LDN), as well. Months later, I am still getting better and improving. It's a good thing I am able to remain on the Gilenya and Ampyra, because both medications have a lot of benefits to them. I wouldn't want to have to be without either one of them. Ampyra, Gilenya, and LDN really seem to work better for you when you are taking all three. It is a magnificent trio of meds. I strongly believe we need a fourth medication, but I haven't seen it yet.

LDN

So after my aunt, who is a nurse, happened to read an article about how low dose naltrexone (LDN) helps people suffering from multiple sclerosis (MS), me and my wife decided to go for it and give the medicine a try. Based on how I feel now, we sure are glad we did. My wife calls it the miracle drug. It is easier to get off the couch and my bed nowadays and my 25-foot walk doesn't take as long as it use to. I am also able to make more errands now and can write with my dominant right hand again. I may write slowly, but I can write legibly again. I can even add filtered water to the Keurig reservoir without me shaking out of control and the water going everywhere else. I think that's pretty epic and paramount for myself to be able to do again. Sometimes it's just little things like that that can make you happy and put a smile on your face.

    What seemed to be winless battles before I added LDN to my other two medications, such as fighting fatigue, being able to go outside in the heat and humidity, and doing things around the house, are now battles and challenges I can overcome every day. I am even able to be in the house without an air conditioner being on and with it being muggy and in the High 70's and 80's in the house.

    Although I still use a wheelchair from time to time to get around the shopping malls and other big places, such as the theme park, I started to push the shopping cart around in the grocery stores at times. This happens to be a big change for me. I would always need to use the battery operated cart with a basket connected to it to put my items in it from the store. In fact, my son would bring it right to the car door for me if I needed to use it at the moment. Good thing places have these battery operated carts, and it's so nice to get help when you need it, but it is also good to have more options and to push a shopping cart for yourself if you can.

In matter of fact, I was pushing a little red shopping cart today while getting some items at the grocery store, and I saw someone who knew me from the dark times before I started taking LDN. She was simply amazed at how well I look now compared to how fatigued and sick I use to appear before adding this life changing medication. I told her I was writing a book to let more people aware and know about LDN, and that I was so inspired by the wonderful changes I am experiencing. She told me to make sure I publish the book as an ebook so that people that can't get out and purchase it, can easily get it and read it on the computer, or even a tablet or other electronic device. I figured right away that that's a brilliant idea. Good thing she shared her thought with me. Besides all of that, she wanted me to tell my wife she says hi.

LDN gradually works and is not a cure, but it sure does work wonders over time. On a scale from 1 to 100, I would say that I feel about 75 these days, rather than 30 like before. My youngest son said it's the best he ever saw me. At my last neurology appointment, the physician's assistant (PA) I have seen most of the time throughout the years, jokingly said the sheet I had to fill out about my recent symptoms was boring, because the sheet was blank. How incredible!

After researching LDN and finding out what it does for people with MS, it just sounded too good to be true. We all know how that goes, because we have all been down that hopeful and dreamful road before, just to be let down at the end.

Ok, so low dose naltrexone gradually works. Does that mean I have to be patient and not expect to see a big change quickly? Absolutely! I am sure you have heard from somewhere, or someone, that patience is a wonderful virtue. Well, it truly is, without a doubt. LDN helps modulate your own immune system, so in many cases it is going to take your immune system time to recover from the long time that you have been ill. This may very well be years or decades that you have been ill and your own immune system has been fighting itself.

My wife, who is also a nurse, told me to wait a couple of months after starting LDN, and see if it's easier to bend your legs and if you don't need multiple naps throughout the day. If it's easier to bend your legs and you don't need to take multiple naps during the day, then it means the LDN is helping, and that you should continue taking it with your Ampyra and Gilenya. Sure enough, it definitely works well for me, and I am gladly continuing to take it with my other medications. Thank God! I really didn't think there was such a drug.

When you feel the way you feel day after day with this horrible disease that sucks so much joy and strength out of your life, you think it'll be alright to wait a little longer if you're going to finally feel better and start seeing results. The chance is worth taking, especially at this point. Many of us just hold on to that hope of having a better day, but after taking LDN with my Ampyra and Gilenya for a while, I am seeing and feeling a lot of those hopes come true. Who would've thought an off label drug could help so much when taken with Ampyra and Gilenya?

I started feeling better seventeen days after starting low dose naltrexone. That's just the beginning of the patience and perseverance you need to have with the way LDN works. It sure is a journey, but one worth taking for me. After those seventeen days, I was now able to stand for a while longer, and take two steps without my cane, or assistance. I know two steps doesn't sound like a lot, but I felt as though I was slowly getting my balance and my ability to move my legs back. Being that we are all different though, I wouldn't recommend taking any steps without some type of supervision. I know my wife and our children were there for me, just in case I needed help. I remember they were all right there next to me and pretty much standing and sitting on the couch with awe and anticipation in their bright and widely opened eyes.

Months later, I am able to be outside on a sunny and humid 87° day. I am actually not forced to be inside where it's cooler with the air conditioner on and draining electricity. I am not even wearing a cooling vest to keep me cool with ice packs in each of the holders. After living so long with MS, I never thought that would be possible again. I figured those days were sadly long gone. I also thought that feeling energy to do different chores and tasks around the house was never to be seen again in my lifetime. I was gladly wrong about that, as well. I don't even feel fatigue anymore. Not on long car rides and not even on hot and muggy days. Am I dreaming?

I am also happy to say I can turn the oven on in the kitchen on hot and humid days now. Sometimes it's very necessary, because the amount of options to make something good to eat requires the oven to be on. This is a big change for me and everyone else in the house. My sons can actually ask me to make a frozen pizza on hot and humid days now, and I am more than happy to do it.

It has been these types of days that I would have easily spent the entire day on the bed or couch sleeping. Wow! What a pleasant and welcoming surprise and difference in my life and in the lives of everyone around me. It is a lot to get use to for everyone. Many days I would just be asleep, but now I am up and at em, and kidding around with everyone.

I actually spent eight hours in the car and a number of hours in the sun at Hampton Beach one day, and still didn't feel tired. I felt great, other than a little sunburn. It was so nice to be able to be outside in the sun with my wife and our two boys. I feel as though I have missed out on so many activities and so much time with the family. At this point of my life while taking this medication, I found myself starting to realize a lot of different things. I find it to be pretty epic, because I am out of the brain fog and can understand a lot more these days.

Although I was the only person in a wheelchair at Hampton beach in the morning hours, I was also able to stand on the beach near my wheelchair a good number of times, and for a good amount of time.

After a while, I actually saw someone in a motorized wheelchair that was in much worse shape than me. The lack of muscles in his legs made me feel so sad for him. You could have easily fit his lower leg in an OK sign you make by joining the tip of your pointer finger to the tip of your thumb. Just when you think you have it bad, remember that someone else out there has it worse. Try and be happy with what you have.

    I don't even feel the urge to nap like I use to every day. It feels so weird to actually do a number of chores like dishes and laundry throughout the day and not get tired. I actually think to myself, "aren't I supposed to be tired after doing all of that work in the house." I know I would have been tired if I wasn't already taking LDN, and that's a fact.

    For so long, I had to break up my daily chores and do a little at a time during the week.

Now, I am fortunate enough to be able to do a whole week full of chores in one day, and still not be tired and fatigued. It feels so odd and so good at the same time.

And by the way, I am back to using regular silverware again. I can actually comfortably use plastic without the food going everywhere, as well. I can even take the shell off a hardboiled egg, too, and flip pancakes and other things over without destroying the food. I still have to use two hands to flip those pancakes with the spatula, but it is a whole lot better than it used to be.

I am so happy and astonished about how well LDN is working for me with the Ampyra and

Gilenya, that I want everyone else with MS to know about LDN and feel better, too.

Even my stride has gotten much longer. It used to be short and slow steps, but now they are a little quicker and much longer steps. It's beginning to feel more and more natural, like how I was the time before my diagnosis. Although I may never feel that good again, I am feeling a lot better than I was feeling before. It is important for me to remember that.

Although I have to get the LDN from a compounding pharmacy and have to pay out of pocket, due to the fact that most insurance companies will not pay a dime, I find it to be well worth it. Yea, LDN is not approved to treat MS, even though it's the best medicine I have ever been on to do just that, treat many symptoms you have due to MS. Figure that one out! This off label medication is bringing my life back with the help of combining it with Ampyra and Gilenya.

In the 1980's, naltrexone was approved by the food and drug administration (FDA) to treat people who overdosed on heroin and had a problem with alcohol. They would take 50 mgs of naltrexone and it helped them feel better and recover.

Eventually, pharmacists figured out that taking a low dose of naltrexone actually helped patients with multiple sclerosis. Wow! What a breakthrough.

Needless to say, most insurance companies will not pay for this medication, even though it would be great if they did. Living the life I'm living now though, is much worth the small amount of money you end up paying. If it helps bring your life back, though, wouldn't you?

It just feels like I am climbing out of a dark rabbit hole deep underground and that whatever improvements I make, even small ones, are actually huge and leading me out of that tunnel.

I remember just clipping my nails being a hard and challenging task for me, but it's gotten to be easier now. I am more flexible now, so reaching my toenails is a lot easier. Even though I still shake a bit, it's still easier to clip my nails now compared to how it use to be before taking LDN. Just like I may need help going up the stairs sometimes, it's still better than it used to be.

After several months of taking LDN, I am now able to comfortably step up a random curb with my cane and not have to hold on to someone's hand or something stable around me.

Although little for many, this happens to be a big deal for me. Slowly, but surely, I am gaining more and more independence.

I was even awake for nineteen hours straight on our trip to Hampton Beach for the day. I sorely recall the days when I would get tired during an hour long drive, but now I am the only one in the car staying awake on a multiple hour ride. Never thought that would happen.

For me, MS is like an off switch to the brain compared to the on switch I feel while taking LDN. So many different things are now visible to me. I can even comprehend so much more now. My mind races so much. It feels so good and so weird at the same time. I am now helping people with words they can't think of during a conversation. That's odd for me, because it's usually me that can't think of certain words all the time.

It's even possible to realize that before taking LDN, you were in a state of mind of being lost and oblivious. You may start to understand and see a big difference between how you were before taking LDN and how you are now. You may begin to see that instead of keeping everything inside of your head for argument's sake, or for the simple fact that it wasn't worth disagreeing with anyone while experiencing MS brain fog, you are now actually speaking up when you see something you want, or when you disagree with something.

Try and understand that this type of thinking is new to not only you, but the people that were there for you when you needed it most, as well. In other words, try and take this change in thinking carefully. Other people are used to how you use to be, and this sudden change may seem like you just woke up from a long deep sleep and suddenly got better. It may be a bigger adjustment than you think. Similar to the way low dose naltrexone gradually works, you will also need patience for the people around you that have to now make adjustments to the way you are, or the new you. I guess things aren't always as simple as you thought they would be all along. It's just so different to be out of the brain fog and not being able to think right, to actually being able to think more sharply all of a sudden.

Don't get me wrong, LDN is not a cure, but it sure does help fight a lot of symptoms of MS. This is epic in and of itself.

For some people, coming out of the lost and oblivious stage may lead to a temporary stage of being found and miserable. You may start to realize a lot of different things you had to go through while you were sicker with this terrible disease. At the same time, you may start to better understand the hardships that your caregiver and others taking good care of you had to go through, as well. Hence the reason why I call this temporary stage of life found and miserable. You now become more aware of how things use to be. It's a very shocking stage for everyone. Definitely not something you would ever expect.

If given the choice of being lost and oblivious or found and miserable, many people automatically say they would rather be lost and oblivious. However, maybe if people understood that a disease is what made you lost and oblivious, and knew the found and miserable stage was usually temporary, then many people would change their mind.

Although it might be hard coming out of that dark rabbit hole and realizing lots of pieces have to be put back together, it's still a wonderful feeling to get better and farther out of that deep dark place. There is now a lot more light in your life. Besides, in a lot of cases, life isn't just a nice walk in the park on a sunny and warm day. Life has many different challenges you have to face and try to overcome. Some more than others. Let's count our blessings that it's no worse than it already is.

After taking LDN for a few months with Ampyra and Gilenya, I was inspired to write this book about how well this combination of these medications work for me. It has totally made a big positive difference in my life, and I hope the same happens for anyone else that takes LDN. It used to be hard for me to get off the bed, a chair, and the couch, but nowadays it's not. Even my 25-foot walk is quicker now.

    I have recently come to the understanding that LDN is a piece of the whole puzzle when it comes to treating my MS. After being without Ampyra for about a week due to the change of insurance, I noticed that I slowed down significantly and became more fatigued. I did not expect that at all, but it happened. I now see that Ampyra and LDN work best together. This leads me to believe that multiple medications are necessary to treat my MS. Therefore, it doesn't look like I will be going off my Gilenya. If it takes three different medications for me to feel better with this disease, then I will be taking all three without a problem.

It appears MS needs to be attacked by multiple medications for an optimal feeling of normalcy, or at least the best chance of feeling anywhere close to normal. One type of medicine just doesn't seem to be enough.

EXERCISE

Even before taking low dose naltrexone (LDN), Gilenya, and Ampyra together, I would exercise and stretch. I knew this was very important and good for the body. I have read so much about the importance of exercise for many years and through many different magazines and other forms of literature.

However, at the time I was diagnosed in the last month of 2004, doctors thought it was a good idea for people with MS to just take it easy. They did not want us overheating and have an exasperation. If I only knew then what I know now.

Ok, so before starting LDN, I did many different exercises for my upper body, but now, I can even exercise more of my lower body, as well. Wow! I can actually feel my legs gradually getting stronger. I am strengthening and conditioning so many different leg muscles that I haven't used for about thirteen years. I'm pretty sure I wouldn't be able to name all those muscles either, so lots of respect and kudos for all of those doctors and nurses that need to remember the names of all those different muscles throughout the entire body.

In my life, I think of the saying that if you don't use it, then you lose it. This statement is very true, even if you have to find it out the hard way.

Although doing exercises in the water is very beneficial for people with MS for lots of different reasons such as not overheating and the help you desperately need and get with balance, I just can't depend on getting to a pool that has a nice regulated temperature. Access just isn't that easy for me. Therefore, I use a stationary bike that I received for free thanks to the MSAA foundation. I also use weights and stairs that I have at home with two railings to keep my balance that I have easy access to. By the way, I also use the counter in the kitchen and a wall in the dining room for balance when I do some leg exercises. Heck, I even use the bed and the couch to do some exercising at times. I guess it depends on where you are and what type of exercises you are doing, or can do. I think it also has to do with the amount of motivation and energy you have and the capabilities that you happen to have at the moment.

The bottom line here is the fact that you can use many different objects and things right around the house. Be creative! I even read about people using cans of vegetables to help strengthen their arms and get the heart beating faster. Whatever helps.

Let's not forget to check with your family physician first before starting to exercise, though.

Everyone is different, so OK it with the doctor first for safety reasons. I have read so many articles about this important step to take before starting any type of exercise. Safety first!

So anyhow, I may not be able to get a good workout by running due to my lack of balance, but I sure can get a great workout by riding a stationary bike. Since taking the LDN in addition to ampyra and gilenya for months now, I don't get fatigued like I use to after exercising, so I can do a lot more these days and go for a number of miles. Usually, I do four to five miles while burning about one hundred fifty calories to two hundred. I use to only be able to ride the stationary recumbent bike in five minute increments before taking a five minute break. Well, now I can do thirty consecutive minutes at level six out of eight. What a difference!

A good thing to remember though, is that we all have to start somewhere. No matter how big or small, as long as we do something, then that's what matters. There are so many benefits of exercising either way. Something else to remember is the fact that if you didn't do anything yesterday, then what you do today is already 100% more and 100% better for yourself. Your body will thank you for it, even if it takes months or years to see results. You just have to keep chugging away and realize there will be days when your body says NO, I just can't push myself to exercise today, and I feel as though I should rest. It's not the end of the world when that happens to you. Hopefully, tomorrow will be a better day for me to exercise, even if I have to do a little at a time. For us MSers, it is very important not to push ourselves too hard and to make sure to take breaks when we need to. Let's keep in mind that every single day is different. Some days we may have the energy to do more, but there will be other days when we feel like we can't do as much as we did yesterday, and that's okay.

Other than getting my cardio workout on the stationary bike for thirty minutes three times a week, I also like to do about 60 minutes of lifting moderate weight and working on my abs, quads, biceps, triceps, and shoulders. I just use a lower weight and try to do eight reps four times in a set with about a minute resting time between each set, and five minutes of rest before going on to a different exercise that targets a different muscle, or even a different muscle group. This way I can get a nice workout with good range of motion. As you well know, range of motion is important for the body, as well as stretching. This helps loosen up the muscles, because we know how stiff they can get with this illness.

Some of the other exercises I do are walking up a flight of twelve stairs and walking back down. Depending on how lose my legs feel that day, I might go up and skip a step here and there. I always have to make sure I am holding on to the railings, though, because my balance isn't too good without those railings keeping me steady.

I also do an exercise where having my foot flat on the floor, I keep my heel down and lift the rest of my foot up, like toe taps. Often times when I am in the kitchen, I hold on to the counter for balance and stretch my calf muscles before I do a set of ten squats, slowly, not too fast and wildly out of control. Slow and steady wins the race, after all. Also while holding on to the counter, I swing my leg sideways as far as I can ten times per leg. I like to do these exercises on the same day I ride the stationary recumbent bike. Sometimes I'm able to do squats and side leg raises without holding onto the counter, but I stand close to the counter just in case I start losing my balance. On Mondays, Wednesdays, and Fridays, I am able to do squats while holding 15 lbs of weights and twisting to the left and then to the right side when I am standing up tall.

Another good way to strengthen your legs is to use a stretching band. I have a band that is knotted at the end so that I can put it in a door and shut the door to do different leg exercises. These leg exercises include putting the other end of the band around my ankle and moving my leg out sideways, forward, backwards, and lifting my leg up while bending at the knee. Lifting the leg up while having the band around your ankle also strengthens your foot and ankle. It's amazing how many different exercises you can do with a stretching band. You can also bring this band with you wherever you go, because it's so easy to travel with. You can also pick up a stretching band at Dick's Sporting Goods or other stores like that if you need to increase the tension. The bands usually come in different colors and different tension levels. So when you think one band is becoming too easy, then feel free to get a band with that has more tension, so it can challenge you more.

    You can also look up many different exercises by going on the web. There you will find many different chair yoga poses and many different exercises you can do with a stretching band. You can use Chrome and type in things such as chair yoga and stretching band exercises. You will be given lots of different types of exercises to do. Try and pick out some that you feel you're comfortable doing. Only you are going to be able to decide which ones are the best for you and which ones you feel most comfortable doing. Just remember to start off slow and to do your best. Everyone is unique in their own way, just try to remember that. Not all of us are like Arnold Schwarzenegger or The Rock, but we can do something. Life is going to pass us by anyway day by day, so just try to do the best you can today.

    I have also incorporated chair yoga. This form of exercising is great for stretching and focusing on breathing. It also helps with balance and helps you become more flexible.

Another important thing to remember is the fact that you do not have to do everything all at once. You have time to do any form of exercises from the moment you wake up to the moment you go to bed. Try to remember that, because it's good to know and can be comforting throughout the day. You don't have to feel as though you missed it and can't do it later, because you
 do it later. You can exercise at any part of the day that's best for you.

You don't even have to go to the gym to exercise. You can do arm circles to raise your heartbeat by either standing or sitting down. You can do two sets of 10 arm circles for each arm in a day. Even once is fine, too. If you are just sitting down on the couch or something, then you can rotate your head eight times clockwise and eight times counterclockwise. Try to do this slowly, because if you go too fast, then you can easily make yourself dizzy. Remember that there is no race.

    Again at a sitting position on the couch or somewhere else, you can extend one leg at a time eight to ten times and then do the same thing with the opposite leg. If you are feeling up to it, then you can do two sets in the day.

    Another exercise you can do while sitting down is stretching out your arm above your head for eight to ten times with each arm. Feel free to do 2 sets during the entire day if you are feeling up to it. It doesn't have to be one set after the other. Remember that you don't even have to do ten to start with. Just do what you feel comfortable doing.

  I know that sometimes we may experience spasticity throughout the night, so before bed, try to stretch your calves and your hamstrings. Whatever part of your body you feel spasms throughout the night, try stretching before bed. Stretching may help prevent the spasms and I hope it does.

NUTRITION AND SUPPLEMENTS

As we all know, eating vegetables and fruits does the body good, and when you have a disease, eating such healthy foods may help your body feel a little better. For just about anyone, feeling your best is the optimal goal in life, in the first place. Eating healthy and fresh greens, such as spinach, broccoli, and celery can help the mind stay sharp. Having a disease such as MS, we need all the help we can get to have a sharp mind, so why not try to consume healthy foods. It is obviously and sadly not a cure, but we may at least be able to reap any types of benefits it gives us.

We have all pretty much heard that eating an apple a day will keep the doctor away. If only I knew what type of apple that would be. There are so many different types. Well, humor aside, I am sure any type of apple is beneficial to consume after washing it, but I am also pretty sure it won't keep the doctor away when you already have multiple sclerosis. Am I being a pessimist or just being realistic? I would say that through many different life experiences and challenges, I am being realistic. Nevertheless, please consume all the fruits and vegetables you can in the proper moderation, and be sure to clean it before you eat it.

Staying on topic of fruits and vegetables, it appears to be a good idea to include many different colors, such as orange for carrots, green for spinach and broccoli, red for tomatoes and red potatoes, white for cauliflower, and even yellow for bananas. This is obviously a rather short list, but I think the point is given. I am pretty sure we can all come up with a nice variety of fruits and vegetables that are more appealing to us. Also remember fruits and vegetables have water within it, so with an overactive bladder, you may not have to drink as much water as you think you do. Usually for good measures, I drink a cup of water every morning before I have my coffee.

I find it a good idea to keep a variety of delicious fruits and vegetables out on the dining room table if you can, or somewhere that's more visible where you will pass by frequently during the day. This way, you may be more apt to grab a healthy snack along your travels in the house. I believe it's a great idea to keep these foods in a nice visual place when you can, because it serves as a healthy reminder throughout the day. You know what they say, "out of sight, out of mind," so let's do the opposite and keep these produce items more visual if we can. In fact, if you can't prepare this healthy food by yourself, then hopefully someone can be ever so kind enough to help you out with this important, and sometimes difficult process.

To help these great and wonderful nutrients go through the body, water is important to drink. You also want to try and limit the amount of sugary drinks you consume in a day. Limiting such drinks will even help you lose weight and be that much healthier. Your body will thank you for it. It may not be easy, but in the grand scheme of things in life today, it's worth the effort you have to put forth. Remember that what you do today will affect yourself for tomorrow.

Another good idea you can do is to visit an allergist. This way you can find out if your allergic to dairy or some types of food. If so, then remember that there are other forms of milk such as soy milk and almond milk, and there are more than one type of produce and types of food. Just try to eliminate what you can't have, and your body will thank you for it.

I also want to mention that I did try the well-known MS diet. However, it just didn't work for me. It was definitely worth the try though, because hey, you never know. Try and then fail, but never fail to try.

You may also need to take different supplements and get your vitamin D level checked by your doctor. Your Vitamin D level may be low, which is common for people with MS, and vitamin D helps modulate your immune system.

Consuming high doses of Vitamin D such as 5,000 to 10,000 international units (IU) or even more has been shown by many researchers to help patients with MS feel better, but make sure you check with your doctor first and do some research.

Vitamin B12 has also been recommended by many neurologists for people with MS to take. Again, talk to your doctor and do some research before you take any supplements.

SLEEP

Sleep is needed for your body to function well, so it's important to get about seven to nine hours of sleep routinely every night. Having MS can definitely hinder the amount of sleep you get every night, though. Between having pain and getting up frequently to use the bathroom, it's hard to get seven to nine uninterrupted hours of sleep every night.

Due to everything that can possibly go through your mind in the middle of the night in addition to the possible pain you're experiencing and going through, sleeping can surely be a big and very challenging quest.

However, as with a lot of issues in life, there are recommendations that may be able to help you fall asleep at night. You can keep the television on if it helps you sleep, but for others, turning off electronics an hour before a routine bedtime may be a good idea to help you go to sleep faster.

There are also some breathing exercises that you can do to help you get to sleep. Maybe trying inhaling deeply and holding your breath for about a second or two and as you release your breath you can count down for a second or two before you inhale again. You can try doing this about three times and it may help you relax more. You can also work your way up to holding your breath for a longer period of time and exhaling for a longer period of time.

Something else you can try to do to get to sleep is to read a book or something like a magazine or newspaper right before bed. Something else you can do to make sure you fall asleep at night is to not have caffeine after about 2 or 3 in the afternoon.

Sometimes having a warm cup of milk with about a tablespoon of honey can make you sleepy. If you can't get to sleep, then it's worth the try.

There is also some Sleepytime decaffeinated tea if you want to give that a try to relax the body.

INTERNET CAN HELP

I'm not saying you can simply believe everything you see on the internet, but through careful and proper research, the internet can be a good place to visit.

There are many great chat rooms such as msbuddy, GeneFo, and even MyMSTeam. Another place to visit is called Healthunlocked and is supported by the MSAA organization. These are great places to visit on the internet to listen to and share stories about MS. You might be surprised about how other people deal with certain issues that you are familiar with. Sometimes knowing what other people are going through can help you and the challenges that you have with this terrible disease. Although it's very sad that other people have to be sick with MS, it's also nice to know that you're not alone. You can also tell people about different things that have helped you on your journey with MS.

With the internet, you can also leave a message for many different editors and CEOs of different magazines such as MS Focus and Momentum. The National Multiple Sclerosis Society (NMSS) is another good place to visit online. This can give you a chance to share your ideas about different topics found in the magazine. Whatever you can share would be great. There is even a magazine that use to be called Neurology Now, but changed their name to Brain and Health, that gives you good knowledge about different diseases and ailments that many people have in this life. Many of which I never heard of before.

It is good that the people in charge of these magazines want to learn about your ideas and suggestions. They are not mind readers and will love to hear from you.

DOCTOR'S APPOINTMENTS

Being that we have a chronic disease with MS, we will need to see a neurologist and make sure we have our annual checkup with our family physician to get the shots that we need. This may include the flu shot, a pneumonia shot, and another shot or shots that are recommended by your family physician at the time of your life. It is truly their job to know what you should have to help you feel better and to prevent other illnesses from occurring.

Even if it's not now, but in the future, I think you should see your physician and neurologist.

I know there are people out there that don't like going to visit there family physician every year, but I think it's rather important. It just may help improve the quality of your life. None of us can afford being sick, especially when you already have an illness like MS.

I realize many people are fearful of seeing their family physician, but I tend to believe that you will be doing more good to yourself than harm if you visit annually. I also realize that there are many people that may not have the time, but taking the time for an annual checkup may actually save time for you in the long run if you become more ill.

There are screenings and tests that should be done in a timely manner. Many forms of cancer can be treated very well when it's in stage 1, and they catch it early. Some cancers are very hard to detect. Especially ovarian cancer.

If cancer is caught at a later stage, such as stage 4, then the chances of safely removing or getting rid of that cancer is probably in the 90th percentile of NOT being able to. This is obviously not good and sad to know that it could have been caught at an earlier stage and prevented from making your body weak and eventually killing you.

Physicians have certain tests they would like to run at certain times of your life, and it will really benefit you if they can run those tests and screen for cancer or other illnesses on you.

Many of us know that mammograms are important. Breast cancer is real. Many people may know someone that has died from breast cancer, or from other forms of cancer. It is so sad, but also so true.

We happen to live in the United States of America, and this country is very advanced in technology, but all of that technology will not help if you don't voluntarily see your family physician at least annually.

One of the reasons that we see our neurologist about twice a year is to keep up on how the medication is working for you and what they can do to better your quality of life. Sometimes it takes a little research on your part and determination. Maybe you can read up on different information that may be helping people that have a similar illness as you do. I am not saying to believe in everything you see on the internet, but I am simply saying that maybe you can talk to your doctor and give something a try. Even if you try it for about a month to two months and just see how it affects you. If you are feeling good being on what you're trying, then stay on it. It goes the other way, as well. If you are not feeling good with that medication, then maybe you should talk to your doctor and stop the medication as soon as you can, but again, talk to your doctor first.

Seeing a neurologist, or another type of specialist, is just important for you in many ways. Sometimes it may take a while to feel better, but try to be patient, because you could be feeling worse, instead of as good as you're feeling now, if you were to stop your medication.

As many of us tend to forget those amazing questions that sounded so great in our head, but by the time we get to the doctor, we just can't seem to think about then. I find it to be very important to write down the questions you have on a piece of paper, or record your questions on your phone. There are a lot of different apps you can use to remind you. Anyhow and any way you need to do it, it's just important for you to bring those questions with you so you do not forget to ask your doctor. We may not be given much time in the doctor's office, so fumbling with questions that you had, but can't think of now, is a waste of time for you and your doctor. All of the conversations you even imagined having with your doctor, is wasted now. So please remember to either use your phone or write the questions down on a piece of paper that you hopefully remember to bring with you when you see the doctor. This can be very beneficial for both you and your doctor. Trust me, I am definitely guilty for forgetting questions I wanted to ask the doctor, as well. Sometimes I think I would forget my head if it wasn't on top of my shoulders.

Like I said before, sometimes you don't realize how good things are going for you, until it's gone. So let's talk about the medications we want to try and how the medications we're on are making us feel. It is very nice to know if there are any adverse reactions we have to look out for. I feel as though we can all learn from other people. Just like we can learn not to make the same bad mistake that they made, or at least try very hard not to.

You have already read about many sayings that I have already written in this book, but I am about to mention another one now. It is said that a wise person learns from other people's mistakes, a smart person learns from their own mistakes, and an unfortunate person doesn't learn from either.

HANDICAP PARKING

I know it's hard at times to park in a handicap parking spot and then walk out looking as though you're doing pretty good and don't deserve to me parking in the handicap parking place. Little do people realize that we have good days and days that are not as good. Plus, they haven't even taken a look at our MRI. Sometimes it's more than necessary to park closer to the store you're about to go in. Just because we may look okay, does not necessarily mean we are feeling okay, especially on the inside.

I think people need to understand that if they see a handicap placard hanging on the rearview mirror or a handicap sign on a license plate, then that will mean the person needs to park closer to their destination when they arrive there. Something else for many people to understand is the fact that there is a lot of paperwork involved in getting a handicap placard or a license plate with a handicap sign on it. You have to see your family physician or neurologist and have them fill out some paperwork for you to prove that you have an illness that requires you to be able to park in the handicap spots closer to your destination. It's not as if you can just walk in the town hall and get a handicap placard or just walk into the Department of Motor Vehicle (DMV) and pick out a license plate that has a handicap symbol on it and put it on your vehicle. I think a lot of people just don't understand the process you have to go through to make sure you can park in a handicap parking spot.

I know not all people mind too much about the handicap parking for someone that needs it, but it's important to realize that sometimes symptoms can be invisible to the eye of an onlooker. I'm sure many of us would rather be able to walk farther and leave those handicap spots for someone else.

Sometimes it's important for us MSers to park close to our destination so that we can conserve what little energy we may have for the entire day. Especially if it's hot and humid outside. Weather can play a big role for people with MS. It's as if we have our own internal barometer. We will definitely be able to feel sticky and humid weather and be negatively affected by it. We can also feel the cold weather. I say this because this type of weather will make us move slower, so it would be to our advantage if we are parked closer to the place we're going.

PROLOGUE

Hopefully reading this book helps you know you're not alone out there, and encourages you to keep smiling and keep moving. Remember everything you have is important, and that things could always be worse. Try to remember that what works for one person may not work well for you, because everyone is unique in their own special way. No matter how you feel, life is going to go by anyway, so try and do your best to keep moving forward one way or another and one day at a time. Some days are better than others and to keep trying to do your best. Bring to mind that if you think you're moving slowly, then try to realize that you are moving a lot faster than the person sitting on the couch.

Something else to remember is to try and surround yourself with good company and around people that will support you when you need it.

It also helps to see a physical therapist (PT) and an occupational therapist (OT) when you can, to help form different exercises and habits that will conserve your energy. It is also important to see a therapist if medications alone don't help you feel better mentally. Depending on how you are, antidepressants may not be enough to help you feel good mentally, and that does not help the quality of your life.

Thank you,

Jim Harmon

James Harmon was born in 1977 in Albany, New York. During his twenty years living in the city, he attended seven different schools and played for two basketball teams while playing different sports. He was able to travel to South Africa and Swaziland after his junior year in high school. He met a wonderful woman and the girl of his dreams in college and they moved to a small, but friendly country town in Salem, New York and would get married and have three fantastic children, but unfortunately their fraternal twin daughter passed away at seven months and six days of life. He later joined the school's PTA and became the score keeper for both of his sons' baseball team after being diagnosed with multiple sclerosis. He enjoys writing and became an author after publishing his first book titled FINDING THE GOOD DURING BAD TIMES WITH MULTIPLE SCLEROSIS in June of 2018.

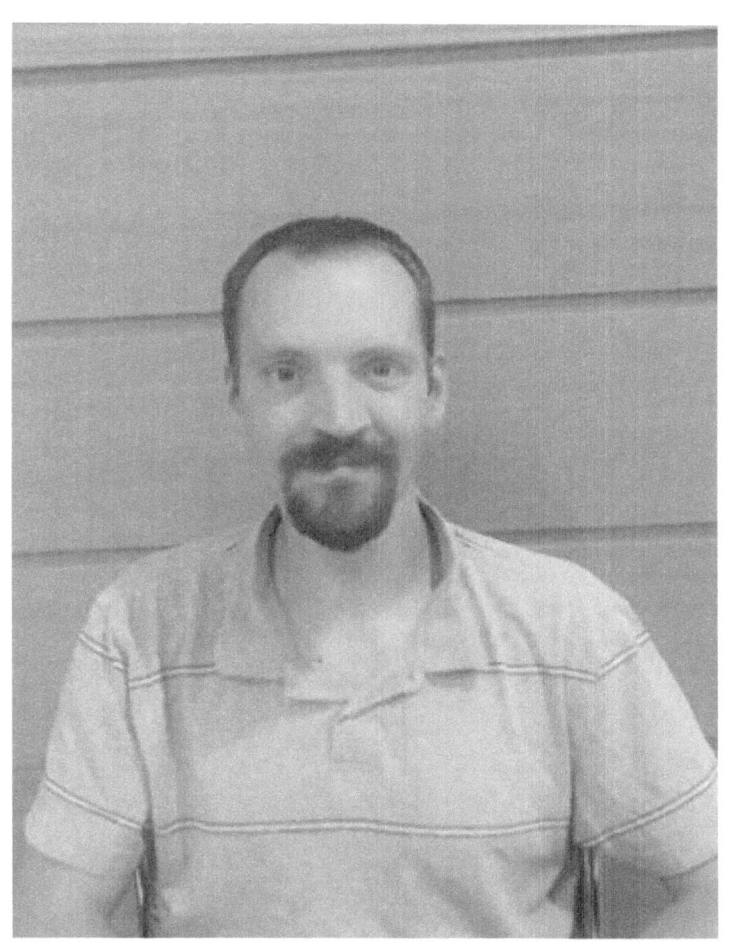

www.ingramcontent.com/pod-product-compliance
Lightning Source LLC
Chambersburg PA
CBHW031619210526
45464CB00004B/1650